Overcome Depression

A Nutritionist's Guide – How to change your Diet and Look Forward to a Brighter, Happier Future – Depression Free.

By Laura Hails

Contents

Introduction

The food we eat creates the person that we become, eat healthy, nutritious food and you will look radiant, have more energy, sleep more soundly, become more active, lose excess weight and ultimately, achieve more.

There is no miracle cure for depression, there are no overnight solutions or magic potions but there is no doubt that introducing small changes into your daily routine couples with daily exercise and the right diet can have dramatic results.

Studies have shown that people who change their diets to a more healthy, nutritious one whilst dumping the junk and getting more vitamin D can significantly reduce their feelings of depression.

This book will explain what a nutritious diet should look like, tips on how to introduce a healthy diet into your life and the foods that you should be consuming more of to help you fight depression.

Chapter One
Depression

What is depression

Depression is a common and serious medical illness that negatively affects how you feel, the way you think and how you act. Fortunately, it is also treatable. Depression causes feelings of sadness and/or a loss of interest in activities once enjoyed. It can lead to a variety of emotional and physical problems and can decrease a person's ability to function at work and at home.

Although scientists agree that depression is a brain disorder, the debate continues about exact causes. Many factors may contribute to the onset of depression, including genetic characteristics, changes in hormone levels, certain medical illnesses, stress, grief, or substance abuse. Any of these factors alone or in combination can bring about the specific changes in brain chemistry that lead to the many symptoms of depression, bipolar disorder and related conditions.

What Are the Symptoms of Depression?

Symptoms must last at least two weeks for a diagnosis of depression.

Depression commonly affects your thoughts, your emotions, your behaviours and your overall physical health. Here are some of the most common symptoms that point to the presence of depression:

Feelings:

- Sadness

- Hopelessness

- Guilt

- Moodiness

- Angry outbursts

- Loss of interest in friends, family and favourite activities, including sex

Thoughts:

- Trouble concentrating

- Trouble making decisions

- Trouble remembering

- Thoughts of harming yourself

- Delusions and/or hallucinations can also occur in cases of severe depression

Behaviours:

- Withdrawing from people

- Substance abuse

- Missing work, school or other commitments

- Attempts to harm yourself

Physical problems:

- Tiredness or lack of energy

- Unexplained aches and pains

- Changes in appetite

- Weight loss

- Weight gain

- Changes in sleep – sleeping too little or too much (Note: if you are concerned about your sleep,

Everyone can expect to experience one or more of these symptoms on occasion. An occurrence of any one of these symptoms on its own does not constitute depression. When healthcare professionals suspect depression, they commonly look for clusters of these symptoms occurring regularly for two weeks or longer, and impacting functional aspects of the person's life.

Also, medical conditions (e.g., thyroid problems, a brain tumour or vitamin deficiency) can mimic symptoms of depression so it is important to rule out general medical causes.

Depression affects an estimated one in 15 adults in any given year. And one in six people will experience depression at some time in their life. Depression can strike at any time, but on average, first appears during the late teens to mid-20s. Women are more likely than men to experience depression. Some studies show that one-third of women will experience a major depressive episode in their lifetime.

Several factors can play a role in depression:

Biochemistry:

Differences in certain chemicals in the brain may contribute to symptoms of depression.

Genetics:

Depression can run in families. For example, if one identical twin has depression, the other has a 70 percent chance of having the illness sometime in life.

Personality:

People with low self-esteem, who are easily overwhelmed by stress, or who are generally pessimistic appear to be more likely to experience depression.

Environment:

Continuous exposure to violence, neglect, abuse or poverty may make some people more vulnerable to depression.

Depression Is Different from Sadness or Grief/Bereavement

The death of a loved one, loss of a job or the ending of a relationship are difficult experiences for a person to endure. It is normal for feelings of sadness or grief to develop in response to such situations. Those experiencing loss often might describe themselves as being "depressed."

But being sad is not the same as having depression. The grieving process is natural and unique to each individual and shares some of the same features of depression. Both grief and depression may involve intense sadness and withdrawal from usual activities. They are also different in important ways:

The Difference Between Grief and Depression.

1 - In grief, painful feelings come in waves, often intermixed with positive memories of the deceased. In major depression, mood and/or pleasure are decreased for most of two weeks.

2 - In grief, self-esteem is usually maintained. In major depression, feelings of worthlessness and self-loathing are common.

3 - For some people, the death of a loved one can bring on major depression. Losing a job or being a victim of a physical assault or a major disaster can lead to depression for some people. When grief and depression co-exist, the grief is more severe and lasts longer than grief without depression. Despite some overlap between grief and depression, they are different. Distinguishing between them is important when it comes to dealing with depression.

Depression can and does affect anyone—even a person who appears to live in relatively ideal circumstances.

How Is Depression Treated?

Brain chemistry may contribute to an individual's depression and may factor into their treatment. For this reason, antidepressants might be prescribed to help modify one's brain chemistry. These medications are not sedatives and are not habit-forming. Usually, antidepressant medications have no stimulating effect on people not experiencing depression.

First Steps to Dealing with Depression -

Get a checkup.

Many long-standing health conditions can contribute to

reduced brain fitness, while not being the primary cause of your depression. Being overweight, for example, has been shown to reduce brain function and can contribute to depression. It may also lower your ability to exercise, robbing you of a key brain- and mood-booster. High blood pressure, high cholesterol diabetes, anemia, thyroid problems, concussions or other brain injuries, stroke and other health problems can all take a toll on brain fitness, as can lower levels of Vitamins B12 and D, and testosterone (in men). Getting these conditions under control can help boost your brain, which in turn will put you in the best condition to bounce back from depression.

Check your medications.
Often people are unaware that their medications may have side effects. In particular, medications given for anxiety, insomnia, pain and even depression can cause mood changes, brain fog, or other cognitive and health problems, so it's a good idea to review your total medication list with your doctor to ensure they're not interfering unnecessarily with your brain function or health.

Sleep.

Insomnia has been shown to reduce brain function, which can contribute to depression. Many people put up with sleep disorders without getting them treated. Not only are both conditions often treatable, but treatment can help reverse the damage done to the brain and lead to dramatic improvements in brain function.

Get moving.

Studies have shown that getting more exercise is a key factor in the fight against depression. Exercise improves brain function as well as boosting the mood which in turn helps lift depression. Walking is the easiest exercise to add to your daily routine. Walking for 30 minutes 5 times a week can have significant effects when fighting depression.

Get connected.

Depression can be socially isolating but making a strong effort to socially engage is brain- and mood-boosting on many levels. Taking a dance class, attending a spiritual gathering, or volunteering helps to engage parts of the brain that are vital for brain fitness.

Eat Well

Diets, which are low in fat and high in Omega 3s, vegetables, fruit and nuts is the best diet to help combat feelings of depression. Adding the Omega 3 fatty acid DHA which is found in fatty fish, to your diet has been shown to improve brain function and also to reduce symptoms in those with major depression.

De-stress.

Stress is a major brain drainer and can be a contributor to depression. Set aside time to think about the stresses in your life and brainstorm ways to reduce them.

Be mindful.

Meditation has been shown to help in the treatment of depression and has also been shown to boost brain function, even in healthy people. Begin with just a few minutes of meditation or calm breathing a day and then work your way up to 20 minutes, several times a week. Yoga, and tai chi are other pursuits that may have mood and brain benefits.

Fight Depression the Natural Way.

There are a number of things people can do to help reduce the symptoms of depression. For many people, regular exercise helps create positive feeling and improves their mood. Getting enough quality sleep on a regular basis, eating a healthy diet and avoiding alcohol can also help reduce symptoms of depression.

Depression is a real illness and help is available. With proper diagnosis and treatment, the majority of people with depression will overcome it. If you are experiencing symptoms of depression, a first step is to see your family physician or psychiatrist. Talk about your concerns and request a thorough evaluation. This is a start to addressing mental health needs.

Diet Guidelines

1 - Eat five or more portions of fruit and vegetables each day

2 - Avoid saturated and processed fats

3 - Eat foods high in fibre and water

4 - Include wholegrains and cereals in your daily diet

5 - Eat more beans and lentils

6 - Eat nuts and seeds regularly

7 - Drink 2 litres of water a day

8 - Avoid refined sugars and flour.

Chapter Two
A Nutritional Diet

Proteins

Protein is a powerful nutrient, it plays a major role in our body, building body tissue and making important hormones. Proteins are made up of a collection of 20 amino acids, these are divided into two - "essential" which are sourced from your food and "non-essential that are produced by your body.

Protein, will keep you fuller for longer, it will help you concentrate, reduce sugar cravings, give you energy and keep your hair, nails and bones strong. The protein in your body is constantly being broken down and replaced. The body does not store amino acids like it does carbohydrates and fats, so it needs a daily supply of amino acids to make new proteins. The protein in the food you eat is digested into amino acids that can be used to replace the protein in your body.

There are two different types of proteins in our diet, complete and incomplete. The difference between the two is determined by its amino acid composition.

Complete Proteins – These are proteins that supply all "essential amino acids" complete proteins come from foods such as eggs, milk, meat, fish and soy.

Complete proteins are great sauces of protein and should make up 75% of our daily protein intake, however you can combine incomplete proteins with complete proteins to ensure you are getting the complete range of "essential amino acids" in your diet.

Animal Derived Complete Proteins – Meat, poultry, fish and shellfish all contain all the "essential" amino acids. Fish and shellfish are a particularly good source of complete protein because they are low fat and rich in essential minerals. Examples include shrimp, scallops, clams, tuna, salmon, mackerel, halibut, sardines and cod.

Vegetarian, Animal Derived Complete Proteins – Eggs and dairy products are also complete proteins, containing all essential amino acids. Examples are eggs, cheese and yoghurt. Quorn – although not derived from animals is a plant based complete protein but as it contains some dairy it cannot be classed as vegan.

Vegan, Plant Based Complete Proteins - Plant-based foods that are complete protein choices, include soy products, quinoa and buckwheat – which are a protein-rich whole grain. Soybeans form the basis of many processed soy foods, all of which are complete protein sources, such as soy milk, tempeh, tofu, miso and edamame which are fresh green soybeans.

Incomplete Proteins – These are proteins that do not contain all essential amino acids, or don't have sufficient quantities of them to meet the body's needs and should be combined with other proteins. Examples of incomplete proteins are nuts and seeds, pulses, grains such as rice and vegetables.

These proteins shouldn't be ignored as they contribute towards a healthy, balanced diet. Proteins that in combination with each other provide the complete range of essential amino acids are called complementary proteins. Complimentary proteins don't have to be combined at the same meal, but they should be combined within the same day as the body does not store the protein it consumes.

Examples of complementary proteins are – rice and beans, spinach and almonds, hummus and whole grain pittas.

Carbohydrates –

Dietary carbohydrates are split into three categories:

Sugars – these are short chain carbohydrates that are found in foods, examples of sugar carbohydrates are glucose,

Starches – these are long chains of glucose molecules, which eventually get broken down into glucose in the digestive system these are found in potatoes, corn and oats, peas and rice.

Fibre – Humans cannot digest fibre, but the bacteria in the digestive system can make use of some of them, fibre is essential for a healthy digestive system. Fibre is found in vegetables, fruit, salad, pulses and whole grains.

The most important thing to know about carbohydrates is that you need them to give you energy, by eating the right foods you naturally become more energetic, you do more, and you burn off more calories. A balanced diet helps with weight control, sleeping patterns and memory and concentration levels. The key is to eat the right carbs and ditch the wrong ones

Carbohydrates in their natural form are good for you and should be part of a healthy, balanced diet. Whilst cutting down on simple carbohydrates such as biscuits, cakes and pastries will increase your wellbeing and help you maintain a healthy diet you shouldn't be tempted to cut complex carbohydrates from your diet.

Carbohydrates are not essential as the body can function without them, however, complex carbohydrates are an important part of a healthy diet because of their high nutritional value. Cut back on simple carbohydrates and increase the complex ones.

The More Complex the better

Complex Carbs are starch and fibre and have more nutrients then Simple Carbs. They have a higher fibre content and therefore, digest more slowly making you feel fuller for longer.

Complex carbohydrates are more filling and therefore will help you control your weight, they also help keep your blood sugars level, which stops cravings.

Complex Carbohydrates you should be eating – <u>fruit, vegetables, nuts, pulses and whole grains, whole wheat bread and cereal, corn, oats, peas and brown or wild rice.</u>

1 - whole grains – these are good sources of fibre, as well as potassium, magnesium and selenium. Choose - quinoa, buckwheat, and whole – wheat pasta and noodles

2 - Fruit – such as apples, berries and bananas.

3 - Vegetables – all vegetables, but in particular, leafy greens such as spinach, kale and cabbage.

4 - Beans – beans, peas and lentils.

<u>**Fats** –</u>

Good fats – Oil rich, nutritious foods like <u>nuts, seeds and</u>

avocados are rich in omega 3 and 6 fatty acids which protect against heart disease, aid weight loss, lower cholesterol and promote healthy hair, nails and skin. Another way to get essential fat is to use cold pressed oils such as rapeseed, extra virgin olive oil, walnut and sesame oil.

Chapter Three

Eat the Rainbow

Antioxidants

Antioxidants come up frequently in discussions about good health and preventing diseases. These powerful substances, which mostly come from the fresh fruits and vegetables we eat, prohibit (and in some cases even prevent), the oxidation of other molecules in the body. The benefits of antioxidants are very important to good health, because if free radicals are left unchallenged, they can cause a wide range of illnesses and chronic diseases.

Antioxidants and Free Radicals

The human body naturally produces free radicals and the

antioxidants to counteract their damaging effects. However, in most cases, free radicals far outnumber the naturally occurring antioxidants. In order to maintain the balance, and maximise the benefits of antioxidants a continual supply of external sources of antioxidants are necessary. Antioxidants benefit the body by neutralising and removing the free radicals from the bloodstream.

Different Antioxidants Benefit Different Parts of the Body

There are a wide range of antioxidants found in nature, and because they are so varied, different antioxidants provide benefits to different parts of the body. For example, beta-carotene (and other carotenoids) is very beneficial for healthy eyes, lycopene is beneficial for helping maintain prostate health; flavonoids are especially beneficial in maintaining a healthy heart; and proanthocyanins are beneficial for urinary tract health.

Antioxidants and Skin Health Benefits

When skin is exposed to high levels of ultraviolet light, photooxidative damage is induced by the formation of different types of reactive species of oxygen, including singlet oxygen, superoxide radicals, and peroxide radicals. These forms of reactive oxygen damage cellular lipids, proteins, and DNA, and they are considered to be the primary contributors to erythema (sunburn), premature aging of the skin, photo dermatoses, and skin cancers.

Antioxidants and Immune System Support

Singlet oxygen can compromise the immune system, because it has the ability to catalyze production of free radicals. Astaxanthin and Spirulina have been shown to enhance both the non-specific and specific immune system, and to protect cell membranes and cellular DNA from mutation. Astaxanthin is the single most powerful quencher of singlet oxygen and is up to ten times stronger than other carotenoids (including beta-carotene), and up to 500 times stronger than alpha tocopherol (Vitamin E), while Spirulina has a variety of antioxidants and other substances that are beneficial in boosting immunity.

Additional Ways Antioxidants Help Benefit our Health

Increasing one's antioxidant intake is essential for optimum health, especially in today's polluted world. Because the body just can't keep up with antioxidant production, a good amount of these vitamins, minerals, phytochemicals, and enzymes must come from our daily diet. Boosting your antioxidant intake can help provide added protection for the body against heart problems, eye problems, memory problems, mood disorders and immune system problems.

Top Antioxidant – rich Fruit and Vegetables.

Blackberries, blueberries, broccoli, Brussel sprouts, Curly kale, garlic, plums, prunes, raisins, raspberries, red peppers, spinach and strawberries.

Plant Nutrients -

The more variety and colour you eat the more nutrients you will consume and the more benefit you will get from your diet.

According to a recent National Diet and Nutrition Survey many of our diets - adults and children - are lacking in vitamin A and

D, selenium and zinc and many women are lacking calcium and iron.

Fruit and vegetables are considered so good for us that nutritionists suggest that the recommended government 5 a day should be our bare minimum. But the truth is that most people aren't even eating 5 a day. Fruit and vegetables provide a huge variety of vitamins, minerals and fibre and if you are missing out on eating them you will leave a big gap in the nutrients you consume.

The best way to get the most from your food is variety. Many people get stuck in a rut, eating the same food day in and day out with little or no variety. In order to stay healthy, the body needs over 40 different vitamins and minerals a day so sticking to the same foods will hugely reduce your intake.

Introducing new and different foods to your weekly shop will not only keep your food exciting but your body will reap the rewards.

Whilst some foods have significant health benefits it is important to remember that no one individual food can treat, prevent or cure health problems, the key is to eat all foods as part of a balanced diet.

Include fruit and vegetables from the five colour groups, red, orange, yellow, green and purple. Different coloured fruit and vegetables contain different nutrients, combining them is the best way to ensure you get all you need.

Many of the naturally occurring chemicals responsible for giving fruit and veg their bright colours actually help keep us healthy and free from disease. Fruit and vegetables contain hundreds of colourful phytochemicals that act as antioxidants.

Antioxidant-rich fruit and vegetables can help to protect against heart disease, cancer, and premature aging.

Red–

Many red foods contain high levels of vitamin C. They contain high levels of anthocyanins which are linked to being effective in fighting cancer, bacterial infections and neurological diseases.

Red fruit and vegetables to include in your diet

are raspberries, cranberries, strawberries, cherries, pomegranate, apples, rhubarb, red peppers, tomatoes and watermelon.

Orange

Orange fruit and vegetables are high in carotenoids, crucial for maintaining a good immune system and supporting cell repair and healthy vision.

Orange fruit and vegetables to include in your diet are Carrots, oranges, squashes, sweet potatoes, mangoes, peaches, nectarines, pumpkins, swede and peppers.

Yellow

Yellow fruit and vegetables contain large amounts of bioflavonoids, which fight infection and reduce inflammation.

Yellow fruit and vegetables to introduce into your diet – corn, pineapple, peppers and squashes.

Green

Green fruit and vegetables contain nutrients including lutein, lycopene, folic acid, zeaxanthin and glycosylates all of which are associated with helping to prevent cancer.

Green fruit and vegetables to include in your diet

- asparagus, avocado, rocket, spinach, lettuce, watercress, cucumber, broccoli, Brussels sprouts, leafy cabbage, spring greens, beans, peas, sugar snap peas, mange tout, cress, courgette, peppers, spring onions, leeks, apples, grapes and kiwi fruit.

Purple/blue

Purple and blue fruit and vegetables are high in antioxidants which promote healthy blood and are believed to have antiaging properties.

Purple and blue fruit and vegetables to include in your diet are blackberries, blueberries, grapes, blackcurrants, plums, red cabbage, prunes, red onions, olives, purple sprouting broccoli, beetroot and aubergine.

Chapter Four

A Balanced Plate

Eat more than just the rainbow - As well as a variety of fruit, salad and vegetables we should also be eating beans, fish, nuts and seeds and good oils.

Beans –

Also known as pulses or legumes, pulses are packed with complete protein and contain almost no fat and are a good source of complex carbohydrates which are essential for good health.

Studies have linked that a higher consumption of beans results in a lower risk of heart disease and developing type 2 diabetes. It is now believed that a good intake of beans probably reduces the risk of stomach and prostate cancer.

Beans are low in fat and saturates and are packed with insoluble and soluble fibre, protein and a variety of minerals. Insoluble fibre helps keep our digestive system healthy whilst soluble fibre helps to control blood sugar levels and lowers cholesterol which means a lower risk of heart disease.

Beans provide potassium a nutrient that helps maintain fluid balance and helps to lower blood pressure. They also contain magnesium and phosphorus which strengthen bones. Many beans contain copper which gives us healthy skin and hair as well as a healthy immune system heart. Most beans provide manganese which is important for brain function and the metabolism of carbs and fat.

Beans are high in protein as well as good source of iron which makes them perfect for vegetarians and vegans. Because they contain both protein and fibre they keep us feeling fuller for longer. They help to slow down the absorption of sugar into the blood which means sugar levels stay even, this is not only good news for people trying to lose weight as it controls the appetite but also good news for people with type 2 diabetes who need to prevent dramatic rises in blood sugar.

Choose from - Aduki beans, black eyed beans, borlotti beans, chickpeas, fava beans, haricot beans, kidney beans, lentils, mung beans, soybeans and split peas.

Nuts –

There are many health benefits to eating nuts, they help lower your cholesterol, lower blood pressure and help you lose weight. The high fat content in nuts make them good for your heart because they are rich in polyunsaturated and monounsaturated fats which lower cholesterol.

Almonds – contain the most fibre, calcium and vitamin B2 which are good for healthy bones, skin, eyesight, red blood cells, nervous system and digestive system.

Brazil Nuts – have a very high selenium content, which is an antioxidant that is essential for a healthy immune system and protects against disease causing free radical damage.

Cashew Nuts – contain the most iron and make them a brilliant choice for vegetarians. Eat with vitamin C rich foods or a glass of orange juice to help the body absorb the iron more easily.

Peanuts – contain the least amount of calories and fat but the most amount of protein and B vitamins. Studies have also shown that people who ate a handful of peanuts twice a week significantly reduced their risk of bowel cancer.

Pistachios – has one of the lowest calories and fat content of other nuts and are the only nut to contain an antioxidant called lutein. Lutein is found in green vegetables and is good for healthy eyes.

Walnuts – are a great source of omega 3, walnuts contain alpha- linolenic acid which the body uses to make omega 3 fats that are found in oily fish such as salmon and mackerel.

Seeds –

Seeds are high in fats that are good for the heart as well as containing beneficial vitamins such as A, B, C, and E and nutrients such as iron, potassium, magnesium, phosphorus, copper, zinc and manganese. Just 30g of pumpkin seeds contain six times more iron then a small roasted chicken and 15% more than a small grilled rump steak, which makes them brilliant for vegetarians and vegans.

Sunflower seeds, flax seeds, alfalfa seeds, pumpkin seeds and sesame seeds are particularly beneficial. Seeds are so nutrient-dense that you don't have to eat a lot of them. Use them in cooking as garnishes or to flavour stews and casseroles, sprinkle them on soup, salads and roasted vegetables. Add them to cereals or smoothies or eat them as a snack.

Grains –

Grains are rich in nutrients and are basic energy foods. Almost all whole, unrefined grains can be beneficial to your health, generally the darker the colour the healthier it is.

Barley – pot barley is the wholegrain version. Barley is good for digestion. It is low in gluten.

Brown Rice – is beneficial for the nervous system and digestive system. It is the least allergenic of all grains. Basmati is perfect for people are overweight.

Buckwheat – is gluten free and rich in healthy minerals. A perfect choice for people who are sensitive to wheat. It is a good source of protein.

Millet – is high in iron, magnesium, potassium, the B vitamins and vitamin E. Millet helps to support the digestive system, improves nutrient uptake and is a great energy booster.

Quinoa – comes from South America. It contains all the essential amino acids and is therefore a complete protein but is easier to digest than meat protein and contains less fat.

Oats – contain more good fats then other grains. They are also a good source of vitamin B Complex which is good for the nervous system and for strengthening bones.

Spelt – like buckwheat is packed with minerals and protein. It is a good alternative for people who are sensitive to wheat, it helps stimulate the immune system and provides a good source of constant energy.

Fish –

Eating more fish is an important part of a healthy diet. Fish is a good source of protein. White fish and shellfish are low in fat and therefore low in calories. Studies have linked good intakes

of fish with a reduced risk of heart disease, depression, dementia and Alzheimer's disease. There is evidence that eating more fish may even reduce the risk of certain cancers.

<u>White Fish</u> – have a significant amount of B vitamins. White fish also contains iodine and selenium, nutrients that are essential for a healthy immune system.

Plaice – is particularly high in biotin which is needed for healthy hair and nails.

Sea Bream – is good for boosting vitamin B6 which is needed for making red blood cells.

Halibut – is one of the best sources of vitamin B3 which is essential for a healthy nervous system and releases energy from food.

Lemon sole and haddock – are good sources of iodine.

<u>Oil Rich Fish</u> – are packed with omega 3 fats which help prevent heart disease, heart attacks and strokes. Omega 3 fats are important for brain cell development particularly before babies are born and in the first few years of childhood.

Oily fish are also rich in vitamin D a nutrient that helps the body absorb calcium which keeps bones strong.

Sardines – not only contain calcium but also high levels of vitamin D.

Tuna (fresh not tinned) – contains high levels of selenium and iron which is an important nutrient for healthy blood.

Salmon – contains good amounts of omega 3 fats as well as being a particularly good source of vitamin E and vitamin B6.

Mackerel – contains one of the richest sources of omega 3 fats as well as iodine and vitamin D.

<u>Shellfish</u> – provide zinc which is essential for normal growth, enzyme function, wound healing, fertility and a healthy immune system.

Scallops – are particularly nutritious, they contain more selenium than either white fish or oily fish and tend to have more iron.

Muscles – are also a good source of iron.

Crab – is a good source of copper which is an important mineral for healthy hear and skin as well as a healthy immune and nervous system.

Prawns – have a higher cholesterol content then other fish but the cholesterol levels in prawns has little effect on blood cholesterol in the body and it is far more important to cut down on saturated fats.

Good Oils –

There are many different types of oils on the market, choosing the right one will bring nutritional value to your cooking.

On the whole oils contain less saturated fat then animal fats such as butter and lard. And more polyunsaturated and monounsaturated fats which can lower your cholesterol.

Cooking oils which are liquid when kept at room temperature are mostly derived from plants, nuts and seeds. They all have a similar amount of calories, which is approx. 100kcal per 1 tbsp. but they differ in the type of fat they contain and their smoke point, which is the temperature at which they start to break down. When the smoke point is reached, the quality, flavour and nutritional benefits are affected. It is important to understand what oils are best for what type of use.

Ground Nut Oil – is made from peanuts and is wonderful for your heart. It is packed with plant sterols that can lower your risk of heart disease. Ground nut oil – as its name would suggest – has a slightly nutty but mild flavour and is very versatile. It has a high smoke point which makes it a good oil to use for grilling or frying.

Olive Oil – is rich in monounsaturated fats which boost good cholesterol and have a beneficial effect on your heart. Olive oil can be heated to higher temperatures which makes it perfect for grilling, baking, roasting or stirring through pastas.

Light Olive Oil – means that the oil is lighter in colour and flavour and it has a higher smoke point making it good for grilling and frying. The term "light" does not mean that it contains fewer calories or fat content.

Extra Virgin Olive Oil – is richer in antioxidants. It has a lower smoke point which means that it loses much of its nutritional benefits when heated. Use it for dressing and sauces that don't need to be cooked.

Rapeseed Oil – is a good all-rounder. Low in saturated fats and high in heart friendly monounsaturated fats rapeseed oil also contains omega 3 and vitamin E. This oil is great in salad dressings but also, because it has a high smoke point it is also perfect for frying, roasting and baking.

Sunflower Oil – is low in saturated fats, rich in polyunsaturated fat – omega 6, and vitamin E. It is a good all-purpose oil, its mild flavour makes it good for using in salads and dressings and its high smoke point means it is also good for frying, roasting and grilling.

Toasted Sesame Oil – is most associated with oriental dishes because of its rich, nutty flavour. It is a good sauce of oleic acid which is good for the heart. Its low smoke point means it is not good for cooking – unless you combine it with another oil, such as Olive or Sunflower oil. It is best used for its flavour in salad dressings or dips.

Chapter Five

Rules for Healthy Living.

Cook from scratch

Take responsibility for what you are eating by knowing exactly what is in your food. Cooking from scratch doesn't have to be complicated or time consuming. look for quick, simple recipes, the fewer the ingredients the quicker the dish, and use good quality ingredients to maximise nutrition. Plan ahead and know what you are going to cook and adapt your menu to the time you have. The recipes in this plan will help you do just that.

Read the labels

Food labels are a reliable, accurate source of valuable nutritional information. Use the labels on the foods you buy to ensure that you are consuming what you think you are consuming. Ingredients are listed in descending order by

weight and include any colour, additives, preservatives and,
nutrients, fats or sugar that have been added to the product.
Whatever appears first on the list is the largest ingredient.
Foods with high levels of sugar, salt or saturated fats at the
top of the list should be avoided.

Know your Sugar

Sugar comes in many forms with many different names, but it
is all the same and has the same effect on the body. Products
with sugar listed at the top of its ingredients list is more than
likely high in sugar. The following are all sugars – brown
sugar, cane juice lactose, maltose, raw cane sugar, raw sugar,
sucrose sugar, invert sugar, glucose, fructose, dextrose, corn
syrup, corn sweetener.

Consider naturally sweet alternatives such as raw honey or
maple syrup or add fruit such as apples, apricots and berries.
Carrot or apple juice makes a great base for vegetable juices
as they add sweetness.

Know Your Fats

Good fats or "essential fatty acids" as they are known come
from nuts and seeds, fish and avocados, they are important
for a healthy, balanced diet. These can also be added to your

cooking by using them as oils such as sunflower and pumpkin seed oil, macadamia, coconut, walnut, hazelnut and olive oils are all beneficial fats that support nerve function, mental alertness, concentration and memory.

Bad fats or saturated / trans fats are known to raise levels of cholesterol and increase the risk of heart disease. These are found mainly in animal produce and dairy products they are in butter, lard, margarine, cooking fats, chocolate, biscuits, cakes, savory snacks and processed foods.

Read the label and avoid anything that says it contains "hydrogenated" or "partially hydrogenated oils"

Add colour

The more colour in your diet the more goodness you will consume. Each colour of fruit and vegetables contains different and important antioxidants. Antioxidants are part of a well- balanced, healthy diet, they will keep you well throughout the winter months by helping your immune system to kill harmful bacteria and infections and they will keep your skin and hair looking good and give you vitality. Vitamins A, C and E are all found in fresh fruit and vegetables and are all antioxidants.

Be prepared

Always make a meal plan and a shopping list before shopping. Consider the week ahead in advance. Think about foods that you love and how you can introduce more variety to them. Don't be afraid to find recipes and tweak them to suit your own tastes you may discover something wonderful.

Consider days that you might be home late or have more work to do than normal and make those evening meals simple and quick or even prepare them at the weekend, or when you have more time, and freeze them so that they are at hand when you need a quick meal. Making your own microwave meals doesn't need to be either complicated or time consuming – it just needs planning. Consider, omelets, stir fries or salads with fresh or tinned fish.

Stay Hydrated

Dehydration can, falsely, make you think that you are hungry. Your brain can confuse thirst with hunger. Before reaching for a biscuit or sweets make a conscious effort to have a glass of water and then decide whether you were hungry or thirsty. If you really are hungry consider what you are reaching for.

Healthy Snacking.

Snacking between meals is a good thing. As long as you make the right choices, healthy snacking keeps your blood sugars level and increases your energy. Snacking keeps your brain active meaning that you can concentrate and remain focused throughout the day and on into the evening.

If you enjoy your snacks, aim for fruit, plain or unsweetened Greek-style yogurt, celery sticks, carrots or nuts and seeds.

Not Just 5 a Day

We all know that 5 portions of fruit and vegetables a day is the recommended amount. Given the nutritional value in fruit and vegetables and the health benefits of them 5 portions should be your absolute minimum and whilst meal planning you should be looking at ways of increasing your consumption wherever you can.

Try adding fruit to your breakfast cereal or drinking a smoothie instead of a cup of tea for breakfast, be more adventurous with your salads, replace your lunchtime sandwich and crisps with a salad and add vegetables to your pasta sauces, stews and soups and before you know it you will have increased your intake of fruit and veg without even noticing.

Flavour Your Food with Herbs and Spices.

Spices have been found to inhibit the formation of prostaglandins – the hormones that trigger inflammatory reactions. Reduce your use of salt and increase your use of herbs and mild spices to flavour your food instead. Use - cloves, cinnamon, turmeric, rosemary, ginger, sage, and thyme all of which are known for their anti-inflammatory properties.

Scientists in India have found that curcumin, the primary active ingredient of turmeric, has anti – depressant qualities that were found to be at least as effective as certain medications in the treatment of depression – but without the negative side effects.

Refined V Unrefined

Always choose unrefined ingredients over refined ones.

Unrefined foods contain more natural nutrients because they have not been stripped of their vitamins and minerals in the refining process.

Fibre

People who eat a lot of refined foods and skip the fruit and vegetables are missing out on fibre. A lack of fibre in the diet leads to digestive problems and blood sugar imbalances. Fibre is the indigestible portion of grains, vegetables and fruit it is used by the body to improve intestinal function, helps to grow healthy bacteria in the gut and helps prevent disease by removing waste products and toxins from the body. Drop the white bread, pasta and rice and increase fruit, vegetables and whole grains wherever possible.

Eat at least 25 grams of fibre every day. A fibre-rich diet helps reduce inflammation by supplying the body with anti-inflammatory phytonutrients found in fruits, vegetables, and other whole foods. The best sources of fibre are whole grains, such as barley and oatmeal; vegetables such as peas, Brussel sprouts, parsnips and spinach, and fruit such as apples, bananas, oranges, strawberries and raspberries.

Chapter Six

Fight Depression the Natural Way –

Through your Diet

Making small changes can have big results. Introduce more colour and variety into your daily diet as well as specific foods known to help combat depression and you will reap the rewards. Building good habits into your daily regime like taking short bursts of exercise and eating well will help you sleep better, reduce stress and increase feelings of well-being.

Fortunately, there are plenty of foods with proven mood-boosting benefits that can help you get happier and healthier with every bite. So, add these happiness-promoting foods to your menu.

Foods that Will Help in the Fight Against Depression.

Apples

Apples are high in antioxidants, which can help to prevent and repair oxidation damage and inflammation on the cellular level. They are also full of soluble fibre, which balances blood sugar swings.

Eat more apples: - as well as the obvious, adding an apple to your lunch box each day, apples can be grated onto your morning cereal, grated or sliced into coleslaw, baked on their own with dried fruit and maple syrup, cooked in a pie or juiced.

Apricots

Apricots may be small, but they're a mighty weapon when you're waging war on a bad mood. Apricots are loaded with vitamin C and beta-carotene, which researchers in India have linked to reduced symptoms of depression and anxiety.

Eat more apricots – chop them on cereal, salads and fruit salads, add them to smoothies or eat them just the way they are.

Asparagus

Asparagus is one of the top plant-based sources of
tryptophan, which serves as a basis for the creation of
serotonin—one of the brain's primary mood-regulating
neurotransmitters. Asparagus also boasts high levels of folate,
a nutrient that is believed to help fight depression; in fact,
research suggests that up to 50 percent of people with
depression suffer from low folate levels.

Eat more asparagus – add it to stir fries, grill it on the BBQ
add it to salads, dip it in boiled eggs.

Avocados

Avocados contain healthy fat that your brain needs in order to
run smoothly. Three-fourths of the calories of an avocado are
from fat, mostly monounsaturated fat, in the form of oleic acid.
An average avocado also contains 4 grams of protein, higher
than other fruits, and is filled with vitamin K, vitamins B9, B6,

and B5, vitamin C, and vitamin E12. They are low in sugar and high in dietary fibre.

Eat more avocados: - Mash them on toast, add them to salads, blitz them in pesto and add them to pasta.

Bananas

Bananas are a perfect choice when you need something sweet and they are less likely to trigger an insulin spike than sugary alternatives. They are also a good source of potassium which studies have shown can help reduce symptoms of depression and stress.

Eat more bananas – mash them on whole grain toast, chop them into porridge whilst cooking, eat them with yoghurt or freeze them and eat instead of ice cream.

Beans

Beans are digested slowly, which stabilizes blood sugar levels and prevent mood swings.

Some beans – such as black beans - are high in magnesium and foliate, both nutrients are associated with helping to prevent depression as they boost the happiness hormone – serotonin. Research has shown that people with higher levels of magnesium in their diets are less likely to suffer from depression.

Beans are also antioxidant-rich and loaded with other nutrients that are good for you like iron, fiber, copper, zinc and potassium.

Eat more beans: - Make shepherd's pie or lasagna with beans or lentils instead of mince, add them cold to salads, put them in stews and soups. Make pates, humous and pesto sauce with them.

Beetroot

Beetroot contains betaine, which supports serotonin production in the brain, elevating your mood along the way. Beetroot also has a potent dose of folic acid in them, which stabilizes emotional and mental health, improving your chances of happiness with every bite.

Eat more beetroot – roast it, grate it in salads, add it to soups and stews.

Berries

Blueberries, raspberries, strawberries, and blackberries are some of the highest antioxidant foods available to us. Studies have shown that patients who were treated for two years with antioxidants had a significantly lower depression score then those treated with placebos.

Darkly colored berries lead to weight loss, decreasing the formation of fat cells by up to 73%—that alone will improve your mood. But berries also carry heavy doses of vitamin C. Too little C - can lead to fatigue and depression. Blueberries are also a good source of resveratrol, an antioxidant pigment that studies have linked to relief from depression.

Eat more berries: - sprinkle them on breakfast cereal, add them to yoghurt and smoothies, puddings and baking.

Blue Potatoes

Blue potatoes get their colour from anthocyanins, powerful antioxidants that provide neuroprotective benefits like bolstering short-term memory and reducing mood-killing inflammation. Their skins are also loaded with iodine, an essential nutrient that helps regulate your thyroid, staving off exhaustion and depression along the way.

Eat more blue potatoes – not always easy to find but when you do bake them roast them and mash them.

Broccoli

Broccoli has high levels of nutritional benefits. Broccoli contains a higher amount of chromium than any other vegetable. Chromium plays a vital role in the synthesis of serotonin, norepinephrine and melatonin – all associated with improved mood. Broccoli is not only a good source of iron, it also contains more than a day's worth of vitamin C, per cup.

Eat more broccoli: - steam it on the side with a sprinkling of mixed seeds, add it to soups, quiches and stir fries.

Brown Rice

Swap some of your favourite gluten-laden carbs for brown rice. Studies have shown that people followed a gluten-free diet enjoyed relief from their depression and anxiety. Brown rice is also high in iron which can prevent the mood-depleting condition anaemia.

Eat more brown rice – replace your pasta and white rice with brown, add it cold to salads or hot to stews and soups.

Brussel Sprouts

Brussel sprouts have high levels of fibre and folate both of which have a positive impact on the mood. Folate helps the brain's production of neurotransmitters. Brussels sprouts also contain potassium, which has been linked to reduced symptoms of depression as well as vitamin C.

Eat more Brussel Sprouts – shred them and eat them raw in salads and stir fries.

Carrots

Carrots are rich in lutein, an antioxidant found in yellow and orange fruit and vegetables. Studies showed that lutein intake from vegetables improved depression symptoms.

Eat more carrots – carrots are great in stews, soups and bolognaise, grate them raw into salads and coleslaws.

Cashews

Cashews are one of the richest sources of magnesium. A low magnesium intake in your diet is associated with depression. Ensuing that your intake is adequate is an important part of keeping your mood in check.

Eat more nuts: - Eat a handful of mixed nuts as a snack, sprinkle chopped nuts onto yoghurt, cereal and salad, add them to your morning smoothie. Nut butters can be eaten with dried fruit, added to baking or spread on toast, try nut milks as an alternative to cow milk.

Chamomile Tea

Research shows that chamomile tea not only brings on better sleep but improves your cognitive functioning during the day, too.

Drink more chamomile tea – try steeping a chamomile tea

bag into warm milk with a spoonful of honey – just before bed.

Chickpeas

Studies show a link between patients with deficiencies in vitamin B6 and those with depressive symptoms. Chickpeas have 20% of your daily needs of vitamin B6 in just 1 cup.

Eat more chickpeas – make homemade humous, add them to curries and stews, salads and stir fries.

Dark Chocolate

Cocoa gives you an instant boost in mood and concentration, and improves blood flow to your brain, helping you feel more vibrant and energized. Studies have shown that cocoa flavanols can boost your cognitive performance. Just a few ounces of dark chocolate a day is all you need to reap the benefits.

Eat more dark chocolate – when you want a piece of

chocolate opt for dark 70% cocoa.

Coconut

Coconut is high in triglycerides, fats that are known to increase better moods.

Eat more coconut – add coconut cream to stews and curries, flakes to cereal and yoghurt or coconut water to smoothies.

Eggs

Eggs are loaded with mood-promoting omega-3 fatty acids, zinc, B vitamins, and iodide, and because they're packed with protein, they'll also keep you full and energized long after you eat them.

Eat more eggs – eat eggs for breakfast – protein in the morning keeps you fuller for longer it also keeps your blood sugars level which reduces mood swings and keeps you more alert. Add eggs to salads and sandwiches for an afternoon boost.

Green Tea

Not only will the naturally-occurring caffeine in green tea give you a boost, the epigallocatechin-3-gallate, or EGCG, found in green tea has been linked to improvements in mood.

Drink more green tea – replace at least one – if not more - of your daily cups of coffee for green tea.

Honey

Honey, unlike sugar, is packed with beneficial compounds like quercetin and kaempferol that reduce inflammation, keeping your brain healthy and warding off depression. Honey also has a less dramatic impact on your blood-sugar levels than regular sugar. Honey also boasts antibacterial properties, helping you fend off illnesses that can make you feel depressed.

Eat more honey – replace sugar with honey, drizzle it on cereal, yoghurt. Add it to salad dressings and add it to herbal teas.

Kafir

Kefir is high in probiotics, boosting the amount of good bacteria in your gut. Studies have found a strong correlation between probiotic supplementation and improvements in mood.

Drink more kafir – add it to cereal and smoothies.

Leafy greens

The most nutrient-dense food are dark, leafy greens they have the most powerful immune-boosting and anticancer effects. Leafy greens fight against all kinds of inflammation as well as extreme forms of depression. Leafy greens are especially important because they contain high levels of vitamins A, C, E, and K, minerals, and phytochemicals.

Collard Greens

A cup of cooked collard greens packs more than half of your RDA of vitamin C, which can not only help you fight off illnesses, but has been linked to improvements in mood disorders, like anxiety and depression.

Kale

Kale has some serious happiness-boosting benefits. Just a single cup of kale contains more than a full day's worth of mood-lifting vitamin C, as well as plenty of potassium, iron, and B-6, all of which are known to help the fight against depression.

Spinach

Spinach boasts the highest amount of lutein and zeaxanthin, high levels of fibre, vitamins A and K as well as other nutrients all of which have benefits to healthy brain function.

Spinach contains high levels of iron. Iron deficiency is a problem many women face and can result in feelings of exhaustion, weakness, and irritability. If you think your diet lacks iron, focus on eating more spinach. In order that your body can utilize the iron you should also be consuming more probiotic-rich yogurt, fatty fish which can improve gut health and help your body to absorb iron more efficiently.

Certain foods are more powerful together than alone. Consuming vitamin C with your evening meal helps the absorption of the iron in your food into your body.

Swiss Chard

This leafy green is packed with magnesium—a nutrient essential for the biochemical reactions in the brain that increase your energy levels and higher magnesium intake is associated with lower rates of depression.

Eat more greens: - shred cabbage into coleslaw, add greens to soup, shred it and steam it and mix it into roast potatoes, juice it with celery and apple. Add raw spinach to salad or blitz it in pesto instead of basil. Add it to omelettes, pie filling or blend it in your morning smoothie.

Lemon

One Japanese study revealed that just the scent of citrus

fruits, like lemon, can improve a person's mood. Lemons are also high in vitamin C.

Eat more lemons – add a squeeze of lemon to your cooking to lift the flavour of the other ingredients.

Lentils

Making lentils a staple on your menu is the first step toward a happier you. Lentils are a good source of anaemia-fighting iron and energizing B-6, and they also happen to be a great way for vegans and vegetarians to boost the amount of protein in their diet. High-protein diets are linked to reduced anxiety and depression.

Eat more lentils – add them to salads, stews and soups, replace the mince in recipes with lentils.

Milk

Perhaps one of the most widely studied nutrient in relation to mood is vitamin D. The relationship between low levels of vitamin D and depression is well documented. Vitamin D deficiency is very common, especially in the winter months when there is less hours of day light. Fortified milk has higher levels of vitamin D which helps in the fight against depression.

Drink more milk – most of us drink milk throughout the day in our morning cereal and in our tea and coffee throughout the day. Try taking a warm mug of milk and honey to bed with you especially in the winter months when sunshine is at its lowest levels.

Mozzarella

Mozzarella contains high levels of tryptophan an amino acid that has a strong link to brain function and serotonin production. Diets rich in tryptophan have a positive impact on the mood.

Eat more mozzarella – use it on pizzas and salads, mix it into mash or top a shepherd's pie with it.

Mushrooms

The chemical properties found in mushrooms oppose insulin, which helps lower blood sugar levels, making mood swings less likely. Mushrooms are also like a probiotic and promote healthy gut bacteria. The nerve cells in our gut manufacture 80 to 90 percent of our body's serotonin, the critical neurotransmitter that keeps our brain healthy.

One cup of chanterelle mushrooms contains nearly a third of your daily vitamin D. A deficiency in vitamin D has been linked to depression and fatigue.

Eat more mushrooms – Add them to soups, stews and stir fries, eat them on whole grain toast for breakfast and add them raw to your salads.

Olive Oil

Studies have shown significant links between the Mediterranean diet and improved mood and reduced depression. Olive oil is the foundation of the Mediterranean diet. Lifting your mood could be as simple as drizzling some olive oil on your salad. Studies have found that healthy fats, like those found in olive oil, were more effective at improving the people's mood than unhealthy trans fats.

Eat more olive oil – if you don't already use olive oil for cooking replace your normal cooking oil for olive oil. Add Extra virgin olive oil to salad dressings.

Oily fish

Studies have shown that increased fish consumption reduced depression in men and women.

Salmon – Low amounts of the amino acid tyrosine in people's diet is associated with depression. Eating more oily fish such as salmon, which has high levels of tyrosine is a great way to help fight depression. Salmon also contains high levels of omega-3 fatty acids, which can help reduce inflammation throughout your body, improving your mood in the process. Research has shown that people suffering with depression, who subsequently had omega-3s added to their diets had significant improvements in their symptoms.

Sardines - fatty fish are full of EPA an omega-3 fatty acid, shown to specifically improve mood through anti-inflammatory actions. Even people with diagnosed major depressive disorder reported beneficial effects from taking omega-3 fatty acid supplements.

Tuna

Tuna is considered to be one of the best mood-boosters on the market. Studies have shown that omega-3 supplementation has a significant effect on mood, and tuna has more than 1,000 milligrams in a three-ounce serving.

Eat more oily fish: - Mackerel, salmon, sardines and tuna are the most obvious choices. Try to eat 2 / 3 servings a week. Eat fish poached, baked or grilled, cook them on the barbeque, make fish pie or fish pate, flake them into salad or sandwiches.

Onions

Onions and all allium vegetables – such as garlic, leeks, chives, shallots, and spring onions, have been associated with a decreased risk of several cancers.

These vegetables also contain high concentrations of anti-inflammatory flavonoid antioxidants that contribute to their anticancer properties. Given the relationship between your digestive tract and your brain, it is understandable why a food that can prevent cancers of the gut would also benefit your mood.

Eat more onions – onions are so versatile, they can be added to soups and stews, salads and stir fries.

Oranges

Oranges are packed with vitamin C, which has been linked to reduced anxiety and depression. Research found that women who consumed two or more servings of citrus on a daily basis reduced their risk of depression by as much as 18 percent.

Eat more oranges – juice it or add it to fruit salads, salads and smoothies.

Peas

Peas are a good source of iron, which can help you combat the low moods that often accompany iron-deficiency anaemia and exhaustion.

Eat more peas – add them to soups and stews, salads and stir fries.

Raisins

Raisins are a good source of iron. One small box of raisins contains 4% of your daily iron requirement, as well as plenty of magnesium, B6, and vitamin C.

Eat more raisins – add them to salads and coleslaws, stews and rice dishes, sprinkle them on cereal and porridge or just eat a handful as they are.

Red Peppers

Red bell peppers—which have been allowed to ripen on the vine - have considerably higher nutrient scores than the green ones. They contain more than double the vitamin C and up to 8 times as much vitamin A. Researchers ranked red peppers as second only to leafy greens as the most potent of vegetables. The higher concentration of vitamins helps to improve your mood directly, as well as boost your immune system.

Eat more peppers – add them to soups and stews, stuff and roast them, chop them in salads and stir fries.

Raspberries

Studies have shown that high fibre intake from fruit and vegetables is linked with lower depression symptoms. One of the highest fibre fruits is raspberries. Raspberries are also packed with vitamin C, low in sugar and packed with antioxidants.

Eat more berries: - sprinkle them on breakfast cereal, add them to yoghurt and smoothies, puddings and baking.

Red Wine

Red wine is not only good for your heart health, researchers have also linked drinking the occasional glass of red wine with reduced risk of depression. Red wine is also a good source of resveratrol, a pigment found in grapes that has been linked to improved mood.

Drink more red wine – add it to stews and bolognaise and enjoy the occasional glass.

Sauerkraut

Sauerkraut is a fermented food and is rich in probiotic content. Probiotics in our diet have a positive effect on our behaviour and mood. A healthy gut has a positive impact on our brain, making probiotics a vital addition to our diet as they help boost our mood.

Eat more sauerkraut – add it to salads or enjoy it with burgers, cheese and picnic lunches.

Seaweed

Seaweed is packed with depression-fighting iodine. Iodine is critical for your thyroid to function properly, which influences your energy, weight, and even your brain functions, leaving you feeling blue when you have too little, and a whole lot happier when you're meeting your goals.

Eat more seaweed – add it to stews and salads and soups or eat moresushi.

Seeds

Flaxseeds, hemp seeds, and chia seeds are especially good for your mood because they are rich in omega-3 fatty acids. Seeds have unique disease-fighting substances and the fat in them increases the absorption of protective nutrients in vegetables that are eaten at the same meal.

Chai Seeds

Chia seeds contain more depression-busting omega-3s per ounce than salmon, and their high fibre content can help you enjoy a healthier gut as well as a happier mood.

Flax Seeds

Flaxseed can be consumed in their whole form, ground into flax meal, or pressed into oil. They are an amazing source of mood-boosting omega-3. Just a single one-ounce serving contains eight grams of fibre, which can help improve the health of your gut, making your whole body healthier and happier along the way.

Pumpkin Seeds

Pumpkiin seeds are one of the best food sources of tryptophan, an amino acid that helps promote the production of serotonin in your brain. Tryptophan can also have a calming effect, making it easier to fall asleep at night and wake up feeling refreshed.

Eat more seeds: - Like nuts, sprinkle over cereal, yoghurt, salad, stews and soups.

Shellfish

Crab

Crab is a serious mood-booster, containing 351 milligrams of omega-3s per three-ounce portion. For people who suffer from depression-promoting anaemia, crab is a particularly good choice; it's high in iron, helping to boost your mood.

Clams

Clams are a surprising source of happiness-promoting, immune-boosting vitamin C, as well as being packed with more than 1000 percent of your daily vitamin B-12. A lack of dietary B-12 has been linked to lack of concentration as well as depression. Vitamin B12 is known for reducing depression in men.

Mussels

Mussels are packed with some of the highest naturally-occurring levels of vitamin B12, a vitamin that many adults are lacking in their diets. B12 helps to insulate brain cells, keeping your brain sharp as you age. Mussels also contain the trace nutrients zinc, iodine, and selenium, which keep your thyroid—a major mood regulator—healthy. Mussels are also high in protein and low in fat and calories, making them one of the healthiest, most nutrient-dense seafood options.

Oysters -

Oysters have one of the highest zinc contents of all foods. Low levels of zinc in the diet has a significant link to mood disorders. Increasing zinc in your diet will help in the fight against depression. As well as zinc oysters are also packed with omega-3s, iron, potassium, and magnesium, all of which have been shown to have mood-boosting benefits.

Eat more shellfish – pates and salads, soups and stews eat shellfish at every opportunity.

Tomatoes

Tomatoes contain high levels of folic acid and alpha-lipoic acid, both of which are good for fighting depression. Studies show an elevated incidence of folate deficiency in patients with depression. In most of the studies, about one-third of depression patients were deficient in folate.

Folic acid can prevent an excess of homocysteine — which restricts the production of important neurotransmitters like serotonin, dopamine, and norepinephrine — from forming in the body. Alpha-lipoic acid helps the body convert glucose into energy,

Tomatoes are a great source of lycopene, an antioxidant that protects your brain and fights depression-causing inflammation. And because lycopene lives in tomato skins, you'll get more of the it if you throw a handful of cherry tomatoes into your salad instead of slicing up one full-size tomato. Olive oil has been shown to increase lycopene absorption, so drizzling a little olive oil on the tomatoes is even better.

Eat more tomatoes: - add it to salads, sandwiches and pizza, stews and soup.

Walnuts

Walnuts are one of the richest plant sources of omega-3 fatty acids, and numerous studies have demonstrated how omega-3 fatty acids support brain function and reduce depression symptoms. Studies suggest that the shift in the Western diet away from these necessary omega-3 fatty acids over the last century parallels the large rise in psychiatric disorders over the same period.

As well as containing high levels of omega-3 fatty acids walnuts are also packed with mono- and polyunsaturated fats which are good for the heart. Researchers found that young men who added a half-cup of walnuts to their daily meal plan experienced significant improvements in their mood over just eight weeks.

Eat more walnuts – like seeds add them to salads and cereals, stews and pasta. Sprinkle them on yoghurt or add them to a smoothie. eat them as a snack with a handful of dried fruit. Spread nut butters on whole grain toast and try nut milks as an alternative to cow milk.

Water

High sugar diets are linked to depression so avoid fizzy, sugary drinks and instead opt for water, staying hydrated is an important part of fighting depression being hydrated enhances people's feelings of well-being.

Drink more water: - try to drink the recommended daily amount of 8 glasses, this includes tea, herbal tea and sugar free cordial. Drink more if the weather is hot or you have been exercising.

Whole grain Bread

Whole grains can improve the amount of good bacteria in your gut, which can have a profound influence on your mood.

Eat more whole grains bread – replace white bread with whole grain.

Yoghurt

Active cultured yogurts are packed with probiotics which are known to reduce depression. The connection between the gut and the brain suggests that microbes in the diet can produce and deliver serotonin.

Greek Yoghurt is packed with more calcium than you'll find in milk or regular yogurt. Calcium can increase feelings of contentment and well-being. As a result, inadequate calcium intake can lead to anxiety, depression, irritability, impaired memory, and slow thinking.

Eat more yoghurt: - eat it for breakfast with fruit and a sprinkling of chopped nuts or mixed seeds. Add it to sauces or have it on the side of salads or curries.

Chapter Seven
Foods to Avoid.

You don't have to be officially diagnosed to know what an overwhelming burden it can be when you are even marginally depressed. Studies show that simple food choices can make the difference between feeling worse and feeling more stable.

The foods we consume can play a major role in increasing the frequency, depth, and duration of bouts of depression, especially if we're already predisposed to experiencing it. Try to familiarise yourself with some of the foods that have been repeatedly linked with mood suppressants.

Alcohol

Alcohol is a depressant, it depresses the working order of the central nervous system which controls how we process emotions. Alcohol exacerbates symptoms associated with depression.

Artificial Sweeteners

Aspartame, the common ingredient that's found in products like diet soda, blocks the production of the neurotransmitter serotonin. This can cause neuro maladies including headaches, insomnia, changes in mood and depression.

Caffeine

Studies have shown that moderate and high coffee drinkers scored higher on a depression scale than others. The reason most experts cite is caffeine's disruptive effect on sleep. Coffee and black tea make it more difficult to fall asleep and to stay asleep. Sleep is connected to mood and disturbed sleep can affect your mental state. Some energy drinks have the caffeine equivalent of 14 cans of soda.

Fast Foods

Studies have shown that people who eat fast food are 51 percent more likely to develop depression than those who don't. Fast foods include hamburgers, hot dogs, pizza, and commercial baked goods. Eating a small portion of any one food is unlikely to raise your risk of depression, but if you eat it on a regular basis studies show that you are at a higher risk of suffering from depression.

High Salt Foods

For decades, fat-free foods have been touted as being a weight loss solution—but many of these products contain high levels of salt. Studies have shown that high levels of salt in the diet can disrupt the neurological system. Not only can this directly contribute to depression, but it can also affect your immune system. Consuming an excess of salt also leads to fluid retention and bloating.

Hydrogenated fats

Anything that is cooked with hydrogenated oils and contains trans fats could potentially contribute to depression. Saturated fats, like the ones found in deli meats, high-fat dairy, and butter can clog arteries and prevent blood flow to the brain— and optimal brain function is what you want, if you're trying to stave off depression.

Sugar

Studies have shown that an increase in added sugars in postmenopausal women's diets was associated with an increased likelihood of depression.

Research has found a link between depression, diabetes, and dementia and that having one of these health issues increases your risk for the others. Researchers have found that when blood glucose levels are elevated, levels of a protein that encourages the growth of neurons and synapses drops. Eating sugar makes your brain work at a suboptimal level—and the more you do it, the greater your risk of depression and the greater your risk of diabetes and dementia.

Trans Fats

Trans fat is the name given to unsaturated fats that don't usually occur in whole foods. Only in the 1950s did trans fats become commonly used in things like margarine, snack food, packaged baked goods, and oils used to fry fast food. Studies have shown that consuming trans fats can increase your risk of depression by as much as 48%. Conversely, studies have shown that a Mediterranean diet, which traditionally uses olive oil rather than trans fats, can lower the risk of numerous health conditions, including depression.

While the author has made every effort to ensure that the information contained in this book is as accurate and up to date as possible, it is advisory only and should not be used as an alternative to seeking specialist medical advice. The author cannot be held responsible for actions that may be taken by the reader as a result of reliance on the information contained in this book, which are taken entirely at the readers own risk.